DIY HE Laundry Detergent

Ways To Make And Use Anti-Allergen And Kid-Friendly High-Efficiency Laundry Detergent

Table of Contents

Introduction

There are different commercial laundry detergents and soaps are present which are highly efficient but cost you a lot while leaving the disastrous effects on your health and the natural ecosystem. For this purpose, it is suggested to use the natural detergents which are anti-allergic as well as kids friendly, high efficient laundry detergents.

There are different recipes which you can follow and prepare your own detergents at your home in less time and use very basic ingredients, which are harmless and safe to use. Along with it is important to take care of the types of clothes and another load you are washing with the detergents and their suitability with your detergent or soap.

Once you pick the ingredients and know their benefits, you can use them in the proper ratios for making the desirable washing cleaners for each type of fabric in your load. In the end, you can find some incredible tips on using the HE laundry detergents or soaps and their quantities for their safe usage.

Chapter 1 – Why it is important to use the DIY HE laundry detergents

In a store, if you walk in a corridor full of laundry detergent, all of the packets, bottles, and container contains marks in the form of a label. Specifically, two letters "h" and "e" are made prominent. They are written with red ink surrounded by white whirl circle along with the blue background.

The words "h" and "e" are normally written together as HE. The HE does not mean that it is only used by males. This is a short form of High-Efficiency washing detergent. It is noticeable that what do these words high efficiency meant for. Specifically, while you are using laundry detergent with HE wrote on it.

What is HE laundry detergent?

All of the laundry detergent with the symbol of HE wrote on their cover must be used in high proficiency washing machines. It may include any cleaner, fabric softener, soap, stain remover or a router. High-efficiency washing machines are may be top capacity machines or front load washing machines.

Their basic quality is they don't require much quantity of water, unlike old customary washers. The HE labeled detergents are unanimously made as a speedy stain remover and are used in low volume water machines. One of astonishing quality of HE detergents is; it can dissolve soil even in small suspension of water in such a way that soil cannot be deposited on clean fabric again.

HE is created particularly for washing clothes in high efficiency working washing machines. High-efficiency washing machines makers suggest using HE detergents. Most of the time it seems that also mention a brand of detergent too.

High-efficiency cleaners are easily obtainable in a top load or front load washers. It is definite by the icon of HE on washing machines. HE detergents are considered best for the use of new high proficiency washers. It is because they are strong laundry detergents used for low water volume in washing machines.

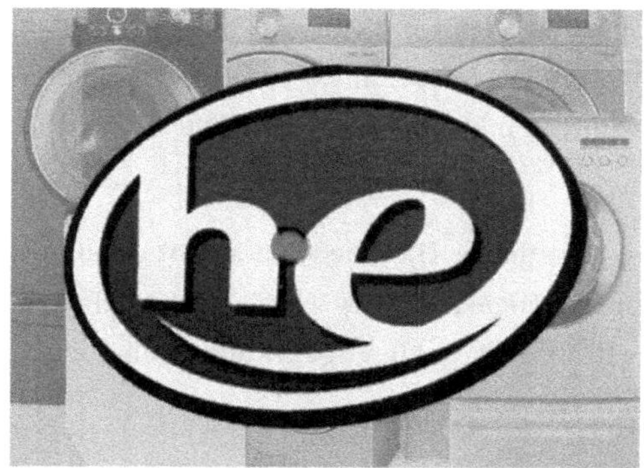

When a detergent gets to mix with less amount of water, with in a washing cycle, it creates an immense amount of bubbles. Even if you use any kind of detergent in the outdated machine with low standards. HE detergent has a specification that it does not create excess bubbles.

If a normal quality of detergent is used in top or front loaded washer, it makes too many lathers. It confuses washing procedure and left clothes unclean and stained. That is why only HE detergent must be used for HE washers. Even HE detergent can work in cold water or other words we can say they aid in saving energy.

As dishwasher detergent will not work, when a dishwasher requires a particularly formed on- siding detergent. Similarly, if an improper detergent is used in high efficiency working washing machine, it will adversely affect the performance of detergent.

HE detergents are certainly available in local markets. The only thing that must keep in mind while buying a detergent is to see HE symbol.it is sold at the same price as other detergents. If you buy them in bulk, it will save your money and ensure you its availability at any time.

In addition to HE, ultra-sunlight also performs very well. "Tide" is very famous brand among laundry detergents. It is safe in use and produces a slight fragrance. On the other hand, the Ultra-Sunlight is represented by HE. It is best for the allergy fatalities, sensitive skin and scent free labels.

Using only, HE detergent in your high efficiently working washing machine with consumption of a little amount of water help empower you to make laundry machines to work as accord to your will.

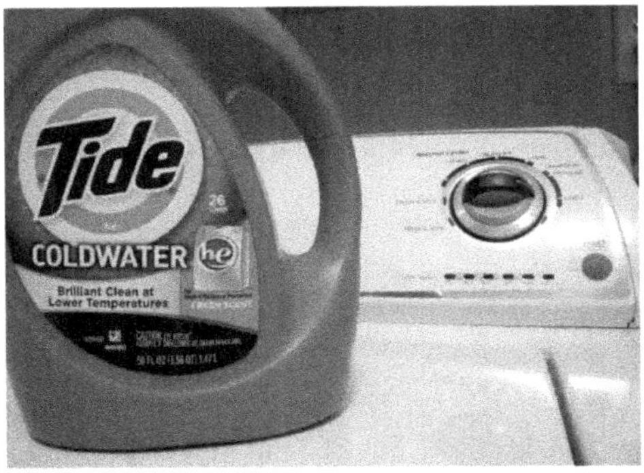

In the beginning, the HE machines contain HE symbol which helps to recognize the use of HE detergents readily. Now a day new sort of machines is introduced in the market which is known as hybrids. Hybrids comprise of top loading styles which are very familiar. There are sensors which mechanically adjust the amount of water.

A most significant feature of hybrid is; it can rearrange the levels of water according to you. Tt means one can easily wash bulk of clothes or even amount of bed sheets. It expresses the qualities of both high efficiency as well as traditional because of certain sensors fitted in it.

One of the leading examples of hybrid is Top load machine GTWN4250 GE. Apparently, it resembles traditional machines, but makers said that they are best for the use of HE detergent.

If a typical laundry soap is used in these upcoming washing machines, then the water level will be raised by the lathers form.it is due to old style sensors and activators.

In order to remove the confusion of choosing detergent for your newly bought washer, you must have to read manual given along with the machines. For the best working and desired outcome of your washing machine, you have to pay attention towards producer's suggestions.

Amount of High-Efficiency Laundry Detergent you should use

Many high-efficiency laundry detergents carry out automatic detergent dispensing. You can read the guide on detergents to know the process of filling the dispensers. Manypeople use either liquid detergents or powder detergents. Don't mix both in one dispenser as it can cause clogging or caking.

 If you select to utilize single unit of detergent packs, those must be put inside the empty washing drum before including water and dirty laundry. Don't place the laundry pot inside the dispenser.

As like all other detergents take time for reading the guidelines and labels about the amount of their use for each load. Much is not always good! If you remember this one thing about the high-efficient detergents, you need to keep following in view too:

• For the normal size of the laundry load, you require just 1 to 2 teaspoons of the HE detergent

• Make use of just 1 or 2 single doses of the units of the detergents for each load. One if enough unless you have a heavy load or is very soiled.

If the HE detergent is not producing the good results for your clothes, don't simply include more amount while washing. Overdose can lead to many problems such as scratchy and stiff clothes, making the odor of bacteria trapped and streaks through the redepositing soil. Instead, you can switch to the good quality of detergents. Obviously, it will need more money, but you will be avoiding the useless re-washing clothes.

Benefits of using HE laundry detergents:

Following are some main advantages of using HE laundry detergents

Effort and time

While preparing the homemade laundry detergents, you should know that this is an effortless and less time-consuming process. Few recipes of making detergents just need few portions of washing soda as well as borax mixed. While some recipes take much time, like the liquid detergent recipes which need melting of some of the soap ingredients and including of the scents. But, the selection of the effort you need to put on while making the detergents isn't much important if you consider the enormous benefits of the homemade detergents.

Washing Machines

Few washing machines need a stable liquid detergent, while there are some recipes of the homemade liquid detergents, which produce chunks of detergent while thickening. Instead of these, you can prefer the powdered detergents which don't produce any clogging in the machine.

Health and Ecology

With the increasing concern about the additives in many famous laundry detergents and additions of fragrance, there can be many allergic reactions which can occur. As well as these additives cause the problems in respiratory system or discomforts in breathing. Few ingredients take a long time to get biodegraded while causing harm to the natural ecosystem. The homemade laundry detergents contain eco-friendly ingredients, which are less expensive and don't produce any unhealthy effects.

Expense

Most of the store laundry detergents are highly marketed, having many additives which make them a highly valued product as well as they are costly, but work which they do is very rare and need much money. Homemade detergents are usually less costly, as their basic ingredients are not very expensive. They don't include any additive and work well.

Chapter 2 – How to make anti-allergen laundry detergents at home

Back in old times, when there were no modern soaps and detergent powders, women and their kids used two things for washing: Bluing and Soda crystals.

Bluing is the dye which is included in the washing water. What it performs is that it tints the white clothes making them a little blue for counteracting the gray shade which appears in the linen and bed sheets because of the extensive usage, while cleaning them and then returning them to their real bright, white color. Soda crystals are also called as the Sodium Carbonate or washing sodas which are used as the washing detergent for the clothes. You can still use these techniques however it is kinds of old now.

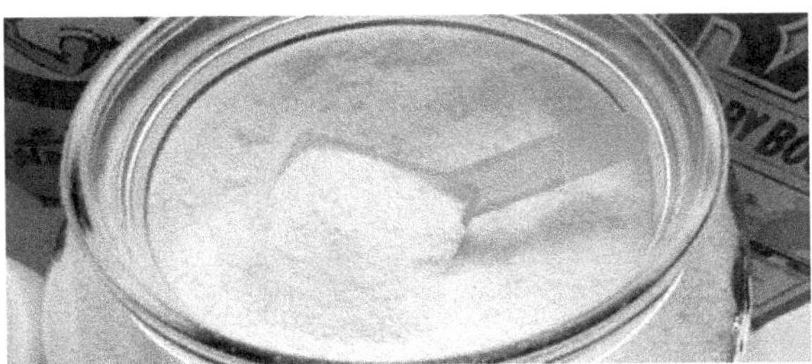

Obviously, you don't want to use the obsolete detergents, so it is better to use the antibacterial as well as antimicrobial detergents, but still, perform the washing in the old manner. This saves a lot of money while improving the detergents (giving the exquisite fragrance) and making you the coolest person.

You may need:

- ¼ cup of oxi clean

- Seven drops of natural tea leave oil (used for disinfecting)

- 1 cup of borax

- 1 bar of bar soap (shaved – this should be homemade laundry bar and antibacterial soap)

- 1 cup of washing soda

1. Shaving 1 bar of the natural homemade soap:

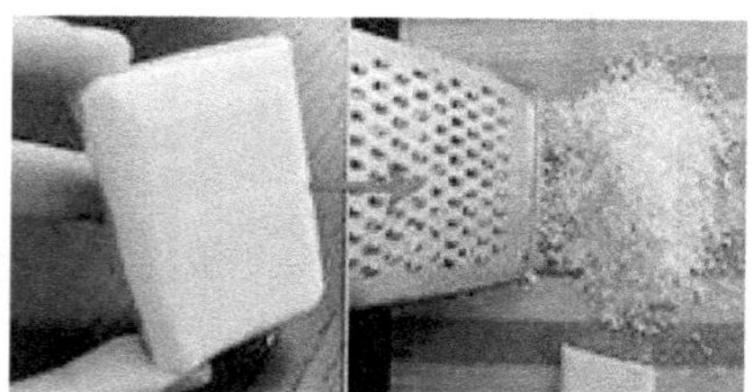

The beauty of creating of your very own soap is that you can form it using the ingredients of your choice with the fragrances which you like. The settings are not hard but need some practice. The process of soap making is quite simple. There are some ways of adjusting the fragrances. But if you don't have enough time, you can get the natural antibacterial soaps from the market.

So, if you desire, you can also blend the mixture in the food processor or a blender for getting the fine powder which gets dissolve easily.

2.   Include 1 cup of borax:

Borax has many advantages. It acts as an important ingredient of a lot of cosmetics, detergents and enameled glazes. Borax is a good antifungal too.

3.   Include 1 cup of washing soda:

Washing soda which is also named as Sodium Carbonate acts as a water softener in the laundering. It reacts with the calcium and magnesium ions within the hard water and avoids them to make a bond with detergent which you use. Sodium carbonate can remove the grease stains easily, along with other wine and oil stains. It is used for neutralizing the corrosive effect of the chlorine and increases the pH.

4.   Include eight drops of the tea leaves oil:

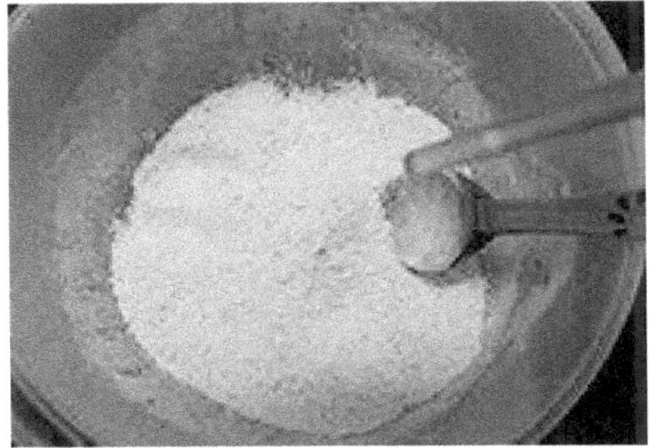

The oil extracted from the tea leaves serves as a natural disinfectant and is becoming quite famous for its advantages around the house. It has amazing disinfecting features.

It can be used for household cleaning which removes mildew and mold, and also good for health. Include 1 to 3 tablespoons of oil for each load (3 spoons for large and heavily soiled loads) and save the detergent in the airtight jar.

Chapter 3 – How to make kids-friendly and high-efficient laundry detergents

Landry detergent is a much easier switch from the store product to the homemade. The DIY products are usually more effective and very less costly. You can prepare homemade laundry detergents which work like the high-efficiency washer.

You may consider the ideas of making laundry detergents at home Firstly, while your friend's mom prepares the ones at home while you visit the friend's home. Once you start doing your laundry yourself, you may experiment some recipes of the laundry soaps. The HE version of the detergents is actually updated take on your actual creation.

Laundry Soap vs. Laundry Detergent

It is necessary to know that laundry soaps are different from the laundry detergents. Soap means something containing the combination of oils and fats along with a base or alkali, which is used with the mixture of coconut and olive oil via lye or water base.

While, detergents are the typical synthetic (at least not wholly) products which are designed for special purposes, like for dissolving both cold water or hard water. Many recipes of making the natural detergents include the talk about the soaps, and they are not very natural.

As the store versions of the detergents, normally known as the laundry detergents, so you need to understand that which detergent is natural for usage.

Natural Detergent (Which Works)

Detergents which are made for working in cold or hot water can clean the inner side of clothes much effectively. Depending on the quality of water, few people may find that the natural laundry soaps which don't work for the clothes well. Others may find that they build up dingy colors on clothes.

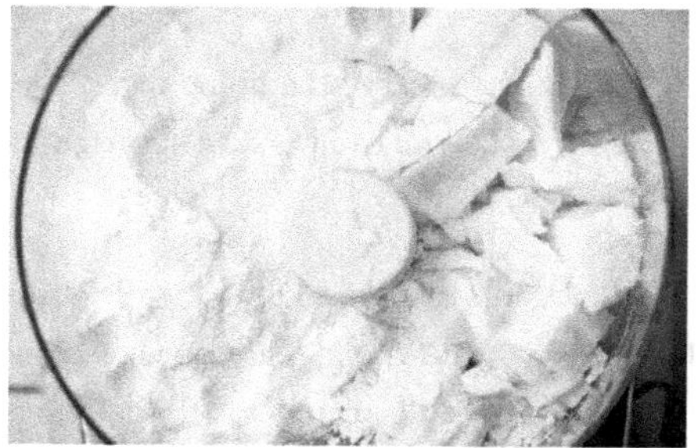

Are High Efficient Detergents Safe?

This is the question which you will see in many comments online. For those who don't win the highly efficient washing machines but know about the friends and readers who do then they can use HE detergents without any problem.

The main thing is that while using the HE detergents, too much suds are created. Thus the low-suds soaps and detergents are recommended here.

Safe Ingredients of Laundry Detergent

Most of the people ask about the safety of using borax within the original recipe. After a lot of research, you may feel comfortable while using borax in the laundry soaps and other benefits which don't come along with the food. Here is the one recipe which lacks borax, but you can search on your own and be sure that you are comfortable with using these ingredients.

Borax-Free Recipe

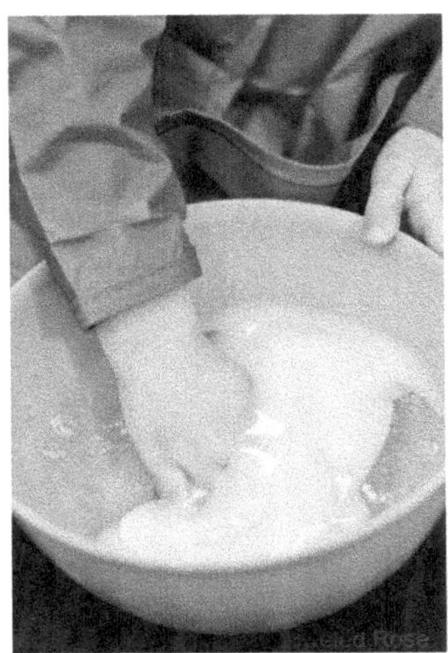

A simple recipe which is borax free and does not need any grating has:

- ¼ cups of baking soda or 2 tablespoons of washing soda

- Two tablespoons of Sal Suds

Just include these during the start of the washing cycle. For an additional boost, include ¼ to ½ cup of white vinegar for rinsing. This step wholly depends on you but seems to be helpful for keeping the clothes pilling as well as look worn.

Why use Natural Laundry Detergent?

As you switched to the natural homemade laundry soaps or detergents for avoiding the dangerous chemicals, colors, additives, and fragrances which are found in the commercial detergents, it turns out that the homemade products are very less costly and are much easier to be made.

Even if you have just started out the natural living and you think you couldn't make your deodorant, the laundry soap can be a simple switch which you can take without carrying out much effort or buying the costly ingredients.

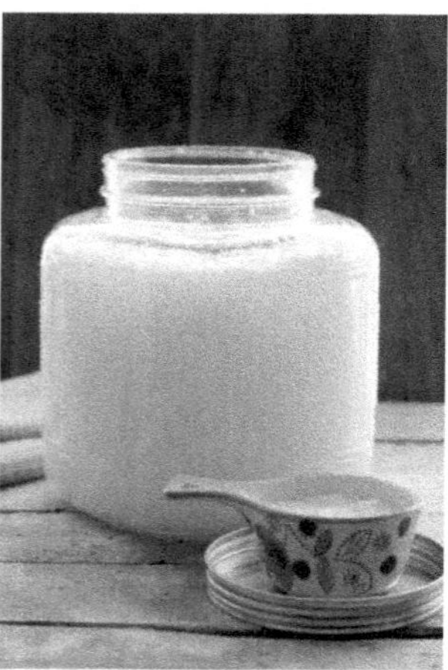

Ingredients of Laundry Detergent

The homemade laundry soap recipe includes three main ingredients:

•   Washing soda: or soda ash, which aids in the removal of oil as well as residue. This is found in many local stores.

•   Borax: is the naturally occurring material

•   Granted bar soap: Just like the homemade soap bars or Bronners, you can use the coconut oil laundry recipe for the homemade detergent. Most of the recipes work well however some has questionable ingredients so avoid them. The coconut oil works much better for the laundry soaps.

Optional ingredients

You can do an experiment by adding Oxi-Clean and other oxygen boosters in your recipe. You may find that they don't perform well when combined in the recipe, but work great if added to the dirty loads of the laundry along with homemade soap.

Another optional ingredient is the essential oil used for scent. You can use lime or lemon essential oil in the powdered recipe, though its scent goes after drying.

Cleaning Laundry

This recipe is made in two different ways: as a liquid or powder. The powder acts much quicker to be created and needs very less room to be stored. However, the liquid form is much effective for the treatment of stains. The liquid looks to be more effective while using it with hard water.

If you presently use the powder form while using other natural products for the stains, you need to pick any one of these recipes.

Ingredients for Laundry Soap

- 1 cup of washing soda

- 20 drops of the lime or lemon essential oils

- 1 cup of borax (or extra washing soda)

- 1 bar of bar soap (grated – it can be homemade or bought from the natural store)

- 1 cup of oxygen booster

How to prepare Laundry Soap?

- Perform the grating of soap with the help of food processor or hand grater. Grate it into fine pieces so that it gets dissolve conveniently.

- Mix the washing soda with borax carefully with the help of spoon while wearing gloves, as they can cause drying if handled directly.

- Include essential oils and mix.

- Store the mixture in an air-tight glass made jar

- For each load, use 1 to 2 tablespoons. Include one tablespoon of oxygen booster if required.

Natural Treatment for Stain

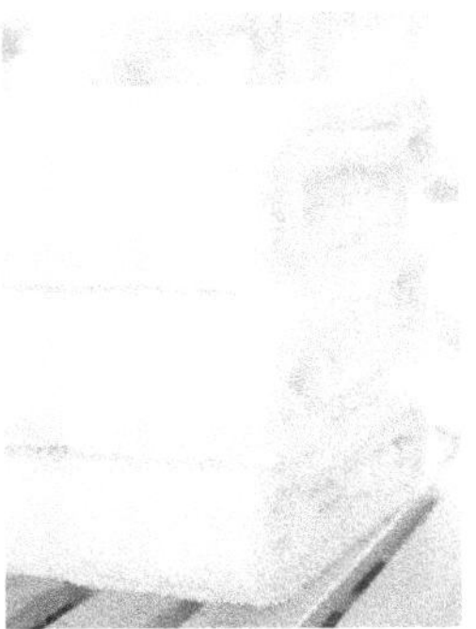

The homemade laundry detergents work quite well; however, they don't work as well as the commercial stain removers or the cold water cleaners found at the store. You can keep a variety of the stain removers as per the nature of the stains. You can keep a small bottle of the diluted form of Sal Suds for the immediate removal of stains which works quite well, even for wine and mustard or red clay.

Bottom Line: Which is better

Obviously, you have gotten confused between among all the options mentioned, so here is a simple way to find out which method suits you best:

Simple Natural Option

This is quickest and easiest way without any extra effort required.

• Include two tablespoons of Sal Suds for each load just like you do for the regular detergents.

• Include two tablespoons of washing soda or ¼ cup of baking soda if you desire to give an additional boost (you can perform this with any laundry detergent or soap)

• While feeling like an over-achiever, include ½ cup of white vinegar for rinsing the cycle.

Cheap Natural Option

If you want to save your money and prevent the dangerous ingredients which are used in modern detergents, make use of the laundry soaps. Just notice that probably don't work

for all kinds of water and you need to do experiment with the combinations and ratios of washing soda for finding what is best for you.

Best for Hard Water or Soft Water

If you have extremely hard water or soft water, then the Sal Suds process is the best one.

Chapter 4 – Tips to use anti-allergen and high-efficient laundry detergents

If you have an experience of visiting any allergist or have an article on the subject of laundry, you may have come across the use of detergents. One of the main steps of allergy proofing of your home is implementing the regular washing regimen – for about each two weeks for the bedding. So, here are some important instructions related to washing as per recommended by the allergist.

You wonder about the simple round in the quite hot dryer will be sufficient for the entire dust mite issue. As per the Journal of Clinical Immunology and Allergy, the drying of clothes at the maximum temperature set for an hour will eliminate the majority of the dust mites in the comforters and blankets. But, the levels of the dust mite's allergens get reduced. Thus, unluckily a simple go-round in the dryer isn't very efficient solution for the dust mite allergic process.

Items to Wash

The sheets, blanket, and other bedding items are the ideal recipients for the frequent wash. Your bodies shed the skin, moisture and oil every night when you sleep. This shows that the dust mites may find your blankets and sheets a home, making the frequent laundering the doctor suggested and wise dust mite strategy for control.

While you try to protect the comforters, duvets, mattresses, and sham, some of the bedding such as quilts, mattress pads, sheets, and blankets may remain unprotected, which obviously require regular washing if you can do. Should the encasing be washed too? This usually depends on the personal preference. The biggest problem is that allergens in air waves settle on the surface as the encasing has the 2-way barrier. Many allergen settings via air will happen on the regular sheets as they may present on the top of encasing.

Regardless of the washing preferences, the encasings will be only very efficient while blocking allergens. Keep in minds that the most encasings of the National Allergy give the lifetime warranties, so wash these encasings as you desire, and never worry about the wear and tear. The low maintenance of Softek encasings must be washed only in case of emergencies. However, you can use vacuum them after every few weeks for keeping them dirt free and fresh.

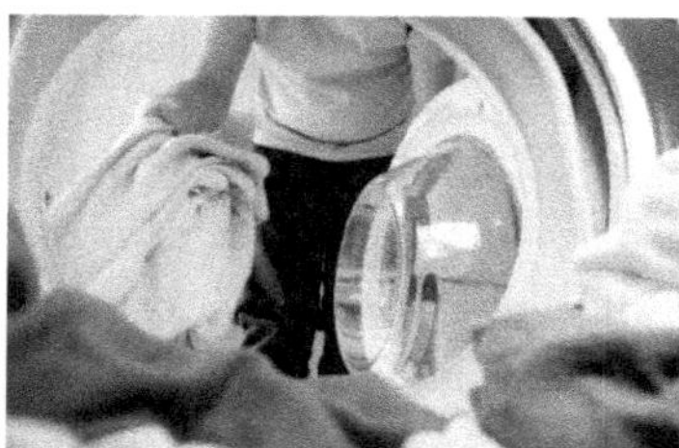

Another important chore is washing of clothes which help to control the allergens. You need to wear the dust and pollen mass while cleaning the closet as if you don't; you will have itchy eyes or congestion soon. Shoes, clothing or any other items put in the closet may collect the dust or dust mite allergen. However, the dust mite allergen can't be the only reason of making the clothes having an allergy risk. The fall and spring pollen can also stick to the shoes and clothes. The pet dander is a quite tacky allergen too which remains on the clothes as well as on other surfaces for a long duration unless they get laundered properly. Also, the moisture of the shoes can promote the growth of mold in few climates.

Some other items which allergy sufferers must launder if required are the stuff toys as well as kid's blankets and pillows. Kitchen towels and bathroom should also be washed frequently at the high temperatures as they harbor mildew and mold.

How to Wash

For the most sensitive items, you can do the handwashing in routine at the sink. Unluckily, most of the sensitive items instruct you for hand washing or the slightly machined wash in the cold water. Without ultra-hot water, items will constitute the allergens. But if you add two tablespoons of the De-Mite Laundry mineral, they will rid the wash load of the dust mites with their allergens.

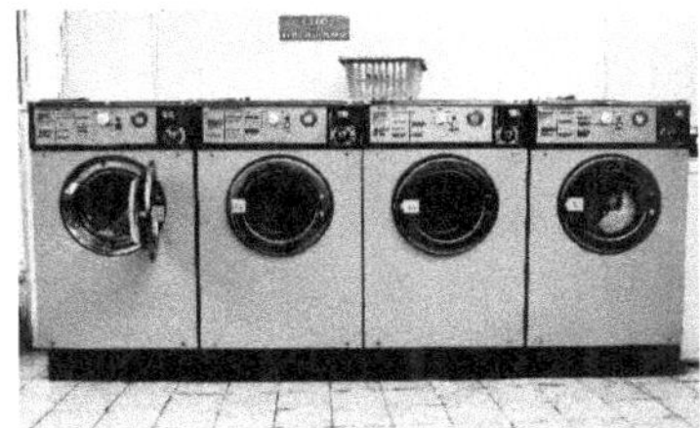

The fundamental design of the washing machine barrel is for turning the contents so a for shaking the loose dirt and let the detergent to pass through and clean the bedding fibers or clothes. As it is mentioned before, only extreme hot water can wash and remove the actual dust mites. But, as the hot water kills the dust mite, the frequent washes of this type may also destroy the feel and look of fabrics.

For avoiding the pit-falls of the allergen free washing, you need to tone down the heat after every wash instead of using the additives for the allergens. The products such as the De-Mite or Anti-Allergen Laundry Detergents are safe for the fabrics and can remove the allergens in both cold and hot water.

The Dirt on Detergent

Detergent is becoming eminent in a very similar way as washers and dryers are becoming known nowadays. Detergents are now available in multiple forms. Such as liquids, unit dose tablets, powders and liquates. They are categorized on the basis of their functioning features. For instance, it is suitable for sensitive skin, shape retainer and color retention, etc.

As a user, you to have wade through many over whelming questions and privileges. The first question which you have to seek out is, either they are safe in use for your family or not. Some people are highly sensitive to certain chemicals. Especially those who with eczema must have to care about punitive chemicals found in most of the commonly used detergents.

Detergents which contain phosphates, fragrance, chlorine, colors and petroleum concentrates must be avoided. It is proved that bleach, softeners, and some local detergent often cause itching after their use. Some of the sufferers suggest that once you have to run a cycle with no clothes in it. Moreover cleaning process must be done twice.

Other than detergents, other laundry accessories may also contain skin injurious components. Like starch, the spray may contain phenol, formaldehyde, and pentachlorophenol causing lungs aggravate.

Sometimes, some residue of detergent accumulates in washing machines just like dry sheets are filled up in the dryer. This is the reason, functioning of dryers is disturbed due to blockage of residue. Most chemicals in detergents are made responsible for causing skin reactions. But according to recent research, it is studied that, dry sheets inside dryers are actually responsible for causing skin rashes to sensitive skin.

Starting Fresh

If anyone really desires to rinse your washers and make them 100% free of potentially injurious chemicals, then it's time to get rid of harmful detergents. And try new chemical free detergents such as enviro rite's Laundry Pre-time.

They are free of lethal ingredients like colors, scents, petrochemicals and another animal residual. For keeping yourself and your dryer clean, it is recommended to use static eliminator which is not- irritating. Also, some washable dry sheets are also available which keep chemicals away from your clothes.

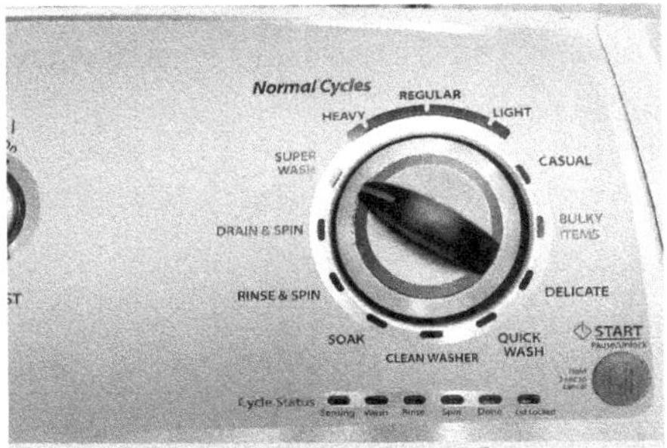

For allergic patients, all in one product are suggested which are safe and clean in use and eliminate allergens. Allergen Allersearch Wash is anti- allergic that contains a surfactant which muddles with allergens and eradicates them.

Some of the anti-allergic laundry detergents forbid dust bugs and allergens deeply by denaturing proteins, so that it may not affect you. These anti-allergens possess fascinating features. As it is used in cold water, can help you to keep your clothes away from damages.

There are numerous house hold items such as salt, borax, and vinegar. They are excellence in removing stains from clothes. They take care of clothes too because they are pure and chemical free items. For instance, adding commonly used salt (also known as sodium chloride) with lemonade will create a stain remover for garments.

Another homemade fabric softener is made by mixing two caps full of distilled form of white vinegar while washing cycle.it will eliminate deposits and scents of detergent left on your clothes.

Here are given some of the valuable tips regarding laundry which are usually unknown to lay person. Although laundry is a bit boring topic to be discussed deeply. Hence it is suggested that using hot water for washing clothes and anti-allergen laundry detergents s best for allergy victims. One more thing that matters a lot is choosing the quality of the product so that it may not cause any damage to the skin.

You must have some knowledge about your detergents and other laundry accessories. Laundry plays a vital role in declining allergens in your home.

Conclusion

There are different kinds of detergents and soaps which you find in the stores for your laundry, but you need to pick the one. For this purpose, you should know the main ingredients which are included in them and how are they prepare. If you think that you can't prepare them at your home by using the natural resources, then it is not true. You can prepare borax free and anti-allergic laundry detergents or soaps at your home, which is proved to be quite beneficial as well as it takes very less time, energy and money to make them.

Moreover, you can find incredible tips of using them and the important points regarding the types of fabric on which various HE and anti-allergic or antimicrobial detergents and soap work. You need to know the techniques of washing clothes too along with the basic ingredients and their advantages. You can try different commercial products too for fast results, but they provide the promising quality.

FREE Bonus Reminder

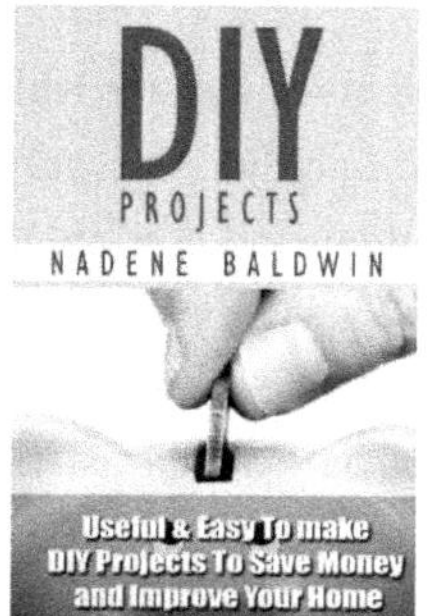

If you have not grabbed it yet, please go ahead and download your special bonus report *"DIY Projects. 13 Useful & Easy To Make DIY Projects To Save Money & Improve Your Home!"*
Simply Click the Button Below

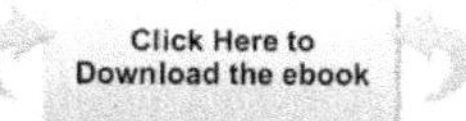

OR **Go to This Page**
http://diyhomecraft.com/free

BONUS #2: More Free & Discounted Books or Products
Do you want to receive more Free/Discounted Books or Products?
We have a mailing list where we send out our new Books or Products when they go free or with a discount on Amazon. Click on the link below to sign up for Free & Discount Book & Product Promotions.
=> Sign Up for Free & Discount Book & Product Promotions <=

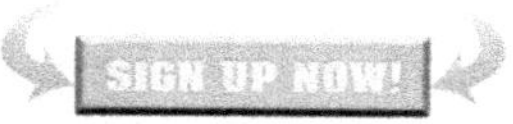

OR Go to this URL
http://bit.ly/1WBb1Ek